Leptin

Delicious Lepti[n]   [Re]cipes To Reboot Your Leptin Levels for Permanent Weight Loss Now

The Weight Loss Solution Series Book #3

By Sara Banks

Table Of Contents

The Weight Loss Solution Series Book#3

An Introduction To Leptin And Leptin Resistance

I want to thank you and congratulate you for purchasing the book, "*Leptin Resistance Recipes - Delicious Leptin Diet Approved Recipes To Reboot Your Leptin Levels for Permanent Weight Loss Now*" This book is part of The *Weight Loss Solution Series* and designed to help you achieve a healthy body and controlled weight loss.

This book contains proven Leptin Diet approved recipes that are not only delicious but also easy to make. If you are on the Leptin Resistance Diet then these recipes are a must in your fight to lose weight and get healthy once and for all.

I hope you enjoy the recipes and good luck with your weight loss goals!

Sara Banks

Are you overweight or obese and always hungry irrespective of how much food you eat? Do you always find yourself eating until your stomach is unable to take any more food? Are you tired of being a slave to food rather than taking time to enjoy the food? If this is you, then this is the perfect book for you. If you have read the other two books in the series, you have gathered some valuable information about leptin, leptin resistance and different ways to deal with the problem. This book goes into detail about the kind of diet that you need to embrace to address your leptin resistance problem. If however, you have not read the other books don't worry because we will still look at how leptin is important in your weight loss journey.

Leptin is a hormone secreted by fat cells in the adipose tissue. Once secreted, leptin travels in the blood, attaches to leptin receptors, and sends signals to the hypothalamus that you should stop eating since there is enough fat. Simply put, leptin is the way that your fat stores usually communicate with your brain to let your brain know the exact amount of energy available and how to use it. When your leptin signaling is working perfectly, your leptin levels will increase when your fat stores are full of the stored fat. This will signal your brain to stop feeling hungry and thus to stop eating and instead start burning stored fat.

However, if there is a problem with your leptin levels like your inability to produce enough leptin, then you will continue eating until there are enough stores to produce the required amount of leptin to signal to the brain that you should stop eating. Congenital leptin deficiency is a rare condition where there are gene mutations that interfere with your leptin production leading to overeating in order to produce enough leptin. This is a rare disorder and normally the treatment is leptin therapy.

While low level of leptin is not good for you, you also need to understand that extremely high levels of leptin are also not good for you. Extremely high levels of leptin lead to a condition known as leptin resistance where your brain is unable to get the signal from leptin when there are enough fat stores, which means you end eating more in order to product more leptin to enable the brain to register that you have enough fat stores. So, how do you end up having extremely high levels of leptin?

High levels of leptin are caused by a number of factors including eating foods high in sugar especially fructose, grains and processed foods. When you have a meal, pancrease normally secretes insulin, which is important in the absorption of glucose from the blood. The muscles, liver and fat cells absorb the glucose. However, a diet high in fructose and processed foods is usually high in glucose after conversion and once the muscles and the liver have absorbed enough glucose, the rest is stored as fat for future energy.

The more fat you have, the more leptin you will be producing and once your cells are exposed to high leptin levels, they become resistant to the leptin. What this means is that you will have to produce more leptin for your brain to register that you have had enough and that your fat stores are adequate. You will continue to eat until you have enough fat to produce leptin for the brain to recognize the signal. This leads to a cycle of continuous eating and accumulation of fat and the only way that you can be able to lose weight is if you address your leptin resistant problems. Some simple symptoms of leptin resistance are constant hunger despite having a good enough meal, overeating, binge eating, low energy levels, poor sleep patterns and insomnia and always being irritable. If you are not sure whether or not you are leptin resistant, you can go for several tests like testing your blood sugar levels or AC1 test that can establish whether you are leptin resistant or not.

We will look at a couple of ways that you can deal with leptin resistance as well as look at over 60 recipes that will assist you to get your leptin levels under control.

How To Avert Leptin Resistance

Once you have looked at the various symptoms of leptin or gone for a test and have discovered that you are leptin resistant, what next? Just because you are leptin resistant does not mean that you will never lose the extra weight to achieve that awesome body and figure you desire, there is still hope. Below are a couple of things that you need to start embracing if you are leptin resistant and want to get back on track to having appropriate leptin levels in your body.

Do Not Eat Between Meals

This is a hard one especially since you are moving from eating too much to not eating between meals. I know we have been told that we need to have small meals throughout the day but the problem is that if you have leptin resistance, you never know when to stop. You will say that you want to eat only one muffin as your snack and end up eating ten until you feel full or your stomach cannot take any more. No matter how much you say that you are going to eat, you are likely to overeat. This is mainly because for instance, if you take a heavy and well-balanced breakfast, then take a snack later on before lunch, you will need to produce more leptin for you to feel as full as you were when you took breakfast, and since you never know when to stop, you are likely to overeat. Not taking snacks; however, does not mean that you should overcompensate during meal times.

Eat A Balanced Diet

It is paramount that you take a balanced diet to ensure that your body is getting all the essential nutrients. It is also important that you take foods high in protein and take foods that are high in omega-3 fatty acids as they are very good in dealing with inflammation, something that you are likely to experience if you have leptin resistance.

Do Not Eat After Dinner

I know we are guilty of taking some potato chips, cookies, or ice cream as we watch our favorite movie late at night or just before we go to bed. It is important that you do not eat after dinner if you are to have any success with overcoming your leptin resistance problem. Normally, when you eat late at night, there is a high likelihood that the energy from the food will not be burned but instead will be stored as fat. Our goal is to reduce your fat stores so that we can get your extremely high levels of leptin in check and not to increase those fat stores through snacking at night.

Avoid High Sugar Foods And Processed Foods

Most of these foods are quite high in calories with the excess being stored as fat. As we all know, the more fat you have, the more the leptin you produce and this then leads to a cycle of high leptin levels that lead to leptin resistance.

Manage Stress

When you are stressed, your body releases the stress hormone known as cortisol. Cortisol is usually responsible for the storage of fat to enable you deal with imminent danger. Any time you are under threat, your body assumes that you are facing danger and starts to store fat. Increased fat leads to more leptin production. Thus, managing your stress levels is important in managing leptin resistance.

Exercise Regularly

Once you find out that you are leptin resistant, you should not move from not exercising at all to like an hour or so of exercise, as this will put unnecessary strain on your body leading to high cortisol levels. Rather, start exercising and build up your exercise routines and strength over time.

Leptin Resistance Diet

As explained earlier on, you need to be careful about what you eat when you discover you have a leptin problem. Your diet is very important as it enables you to address the problem slowly over time and as you do so, you learn how to eat more healthy foods. It is important that as you start on a leptin resistance diet, you know what to eat and what to avoid. We will have a look at some of these foods to enable you make better decisions.

What You Can Eat

Your diet should comprise of mostly vegetables and proteins with a little carbohydrates and fruit since most fruits are high in fructose (natural sugar). Below is a list of all the foods that you can eat:

Nuts: Almonds, Cashews, Macadamia, Hazelnuts, Pecans, Walnuts

Fish: Halibut, Herring, Tuna, Sardines, Cod, Crab, Lobster, Oysters, Salmon, Sardines, Scallops, Shrimp, Tilapia

Poultry: Chicken and Turkey with no skin

Dairy: Goat cheese, no-fat cottage cheese, no-fat ricotta cheese, no-fat cream cheese, feta cheese and Parmesan cheese

Vegetables: Zucchini, watercress, turnip, sprouts, spinach, snow peas, scallions, rutabaga, radishes, parsley, onions, mushroom, leeks, kale, lettuce, fennel, eggplant, cilantro, chives, chard, celery, cauliflower, cabbage, broccoli, bok choy, asparagus, arugula, bell peppers and artichoke hearts

Fruits: Apples, apricots, strawberries, blueberries, avocado, olives, nectarines, kiwi, grapefruit, cherries, peaches, pears, raspberries and plums

Ensure that you limit your intake of fruit owing to its high fructose levels.

Carbohydrates: Eat more of starchy vegetables and whole grain foods that are high in fiber like manna from heaven bread.

Fats and oils: Use avocado oil and olive oil mostly while using coconut oil, sesame oil and butter in limited quantities.

Use sweeteners like stevia in limited quantities.

You can use all spices.

You can have desserts like twice a week or even less times. You can instead opt for smoothies occasionally if you want something sweet but healthy.

What To Avoid Or At Least Reduce Intake

While it can be hard to list all the foods you should try to avoid or reduce their intake, your guide should be to focus more on eating whole foods, vegetables and fruits while reducing your intake of starchy foods, foods high in sugar as well as processed foods. While it is advisable to take fruit, try not to overdo the fruits, as some are quite high in fructose.

Dairy: Milk, Ice cream, Cheddar cheese, Swiss cheese

Legumes: Peanut butter, peanuts, chickpeas, lima beans, pinto beans

Vegetables: Yam, pumpkin

Snack foods: chips, cakes, energy bars, candy, cookies, breakfast bars

Sugar and Artificial sweeteners: maple syrup, corn syrup, fructose, honey

Fruits high in fructose like dried fruit, cantaloupe, muffins and waffles

All fried foods

Breakfast Recipes

Rosemary Eggs

Makes 2 Servings

Ingredients

2 eggs

½ teaspoon chopped fresh rosemary

3 tablespoons low-fat cream cheese

1 tablespoon fresh lemon juice

1 teaspoon avocado oil

1 teaspoon flax oil

1 ripe avocado

Pinch of cayenne

Salt to taste

2 slices of manna from heaven bread

Instructions

Mix the fresh rosemary, cheese, lemon juice, avocado oil, flax oil, salt and a pinch of cayenne on a bowl using a fork.

In a deep pan, add about two inches of water, bring to boil then simmer.

Crack the eggs one at a time in a cup and mix then slowly slip the egg mixture into the water as close to the surface as possible. Simmer the eggs for five minutes then remove using a slotted spoon and drain off using excess water.

You can then toast your bread. Cut the avocado into two then remove the seed and cut the meat with the skin on, then scoop the chopped avocado onto your toasted bread. Top the bread and avocado with the poached eggs and cheese mixture.

Hard-Boiled Eggs With Spinach

Makes 2 Servings

Ingredients

1 cup baby spinach

2 eggs

3 tablespoons flax oil

2 tablespoons sesame seeds

½ cup chopped fresh basil

1 teaspoon tamari

1 tablespoon flax seeds

Pinch of cinnamon

Instructions

For the dressing, mix the flax oil, sesame seeds, basil, tamari, flax seeds and cinnamon in a blender. Place the eggs in a saucepan, cover with cold water. Bring to boil and reduce the heat and simmer for 5 minutes.

Fill a saucepan 1/3 full with water, and bring to a boil then put the spinach and turn down to simmer for five minutes.

Cool the eggs in cold water peel and slice them. Drain your baby spinach and divide between two plates.

Arrange the sliced eggs on top of the spinach and drizzle with the dressing.

Zucchini Pancakes

Makes 1 Serving

Ingredients

¼ cup fat-free cottage cheese

1 egg white

2/3 cup shredded zucchini

1 tablespoon whole wheat flour

1 tablespoon olive oil

1 tablespoon minced onion

Garlic powder and salt to taste

Instructions

Preheat a non-stick pan over medium heat. Mix all ingredients in a bowl except the egg white. Beat the egg white until stiff and fold egg into the zucchini mixture.

Spread the batter onto the pan and spread out. Let it cook until batter sets before turning.

Avocado And Smoked Almond Toasts

Makes 2 Servings

Ingredients

1 ripe avocado

6 ounces smoked salmon

1 garlic, chopped

¼ cup chopped fresh cilantro

2 slices manna from heaven bread

1 teaspoon flax oil

1 tablespoon lemon juice

Instructions

Put the avocado, garlic, lemon juice, cilantro and flax oil in a blender and blend.

Toast the two slices of bread then add the avocado and top with the smoked salmon.

Boiled Eggs With Bread

Makes 2 Servings

Ingredients

2 slices of manna from heaven bread

2 eggs

Pinch of cayenne

Salt to taste

Instructions

Place eggs in a saucepan, cover with cold water and bring to boil, then reduce the heat and simmer for three minutes.

Cool the eggs in cold water then remove the shells. Cut the eggs into large pieces and put on each piece of bread then sprinkle with cayenne and salt.

Raspberry Vanilla Oatmeal

Makes 2 Servings

Ingredients

¾ cup uncooked oats

Fresh raspberries to taste

½ cup almond milk

½ scoop of whey protein powder

2 dates blended in water

½ teaspoon vanilla extract

Walnuts or almonds to garnish

A dash of salt

Instructions

Mix the ingredients except the nuts and refrigerate overnight.

Serve cold or warm and top with the raspberries and nuts.

Turkey Sausage With Poached Eggs

Makes 2 Servings

Ingredients

2 turkey sausages

2 poached eggs

Pinch of cayenne

Salt to taste

Instructions

Broil the sausages for five minutes on each side, blot excess oil with paper towels and put on a plate.

Top with poached eggs sprinkled with eggs and cayenne pepper.

Scrambled Tofu

Makes 4 Servings

Ingredients

1 lb firm tofu

½ teaspoon turmeric

2 tablespoons nutritional yeast

2 teaspoons low sodium tamari

1/8 teaspoon black pepper

1/8 teaspoon cayenne pepper

½ bell pepper diced

1 broccoli stalk, chopped

½ onion diced

1 tablespoon canola oil

2 slices bacon

Instructions

Drain the tofu and cut into small pieces in a mixing bowl. Add the tamari, turmeric, yeast, pepper and cayenne. Using a fork mash it all up until there are no large chunks; you can use this immediately or cover with plastic wrap and refrigerate overnight.

Heat the canola oil in a frying pan then add the bacon and sauté until brown and crispy. Add the vegetables and stir-fry until tender. Finally, add the tofu mixture and stir-fry until the tofu is heated through.

Mushroom And Onion Frittata

Makes 2 Servings

Ingredients

1 lb sliced fresh mushrooms

3 tablespoons butter

1 red onion, chopped

1 shallot, chopped

3 tablespoons olive oil

¼ cup shredded feta cheese

¼ cup shredded Parmesan cheese

8 eggs

¼ teaspoon pepper

¼ teaspoon salt

Instructions

Sauté mushrooms, onions and butter in oil in an ovenproof pan. Reduce heat to medium and cook for 20 minutes until golden brown while stirring occasionally. Add the garlic and shallot and cook for one minute longer. Reduce the heat then sprinkle the cheeses and then whisk the eggs, salt and pepper in a bowl and pour on top. Cover and cook for five minutes until eggs are set.

Uncover the skillet and cook for 3-4 minutes or until eggs are completely set. Allow it to cool for five minutes then cut into wedges.

Avocado And Ham Scramble

Makes 4 Servings

Ingredients

8 eggs

1 teaspoon garlic powder

¼ cup fat-free milk

¼ teaspoon pepper

1 tablespoon butter

1 ripe avocado, peeled and cubed

1 cup cooked ham, cubed

½ cup shredded Parmesan Cheese

Instructions

Whisk the eggs, garlic powder, milk and pepper in a bowl then stir in ham. Melt butter in a large pan over medium heat. Add the egg mixture and cook until almost set then add the avocado and cheese. Stir and cook until set.

Deviled Eggs

Makes 1 Serving

2 hard-boiled eggs

1 tablespoons non-fat cottage cheese

1 teaspoon chopped parsley

1 teaspoon mustard

Paprika as garnish

Instructions

Peel the eggs, slice lengthwise, and remove the yolks.

Put the yolks, cheese, mustard, salt, parsley, and pepper in a mixing bowl.

Mash with a folk until blended then return yolks to egg white and garnish with parsley and paprika.

Lunch Recipes

Chicken Salad

Makes 2 Servings

Ingredients

1 boneless, skinless chicken breast

¼ cup chopped walnuts

1 head romaine lettuce, washed and dried

1 ripe avocado

6 kalamata olives, halved and pitted

For the dressing

¼ cup extra virgin olive oil

1 garlic clove

Salt to taste

¼ teaspoon Dijon mustard

2 tablespoons red wine vinegar

Instructions

Mix the dressing ingredients in a blender.

Bring 2 inches of water to a boil in a deep pan, reduce to simmer and add the chicken breasts and simmer for 10-15 minutes.

Combine the lettuce, walnuts, avocado and olives in a bowl. Add half of the dressing to the salad and toss well then divide between two plates. Slice the chicken diagonally and arrange on the salad on the two plates.

Drizzle more dressing on each chicken and serve.

Baked Salmon And Asparagus

Makes 2 Servings

Ingredients

1 tablespoon avocado oil

2 (6-ounce) salmon fillets

¾ lb asparagus

Marinade

½ cup extra virgin olive oil

¼ cup fresh lemon juice

1/3 cup chopped dill

Pinch of black pepper

¼ teaspoon salt

Pinch of cayenne

Instructions

Preheat the oven to 400ºF. Combine the marinade ingredients in a blender. Place the salmon, skin side up in a glass baking dish and cover with the marinade. Refrigerate for at least an hour.

Bake for five minutes, turn over, and bake for another five minutes.

Fill a deep pan with 1 ½ inches of water. Bring to boil and drop the asparagus. Simmer for five minutes, drain and drizzle avocado oil on top. Add pepper and salt to taste.

Citrus Chicken Salad

Makes 2 Servings

Ingredients

2 cooked chicken breast halves, cubed

1 cucumber, peeled and chopped

2 celery stalks, chopped

1 tablespoon minced parsley

½ avocado, pitted and chopped

¼ cup chopped walnuts

½ red bell pepper

2 tablespoons chopped cilantro

Dressing

1 tablespoon fresh dill

1 tablespoon olive oil

1 tablespoon minced parsley

3 tablespoons sesame oil

Salt and pepper to taste

Zest of one orange

Instructions

Mix the walnuts, bell pepper, avocado, parsley, cilantro, cucumber, celery stalks and cooked chicken.

Combine the dressing ingredients in another bowl and mix using a wire whisk.

Pour the dressing over the chicken mixture and store covered in the fridge for a day to let the flavors to blend.

Serve this with a green salad.

Romaine Salad

Makes 3 Servings

Ingredients

3 cups romaine lettuce, washed and dried

1 celery stalk chopped

½ cup pecans

1 small head radicchio washed and sliced

½ yellow bell pepper, cut into strips

Vinaigrette

¼ cup fresh chopped mint

¼ cup extra virgin olive oil

1 tablespoon lime juice

2 tablespoons lemon juice

Instructions

Mix the vinaigrette ingredients in a blender. Put the other ingredients in a bowl and pour the dressing. Serve.

Asparagus Soup And Deviled Eggs

Makes 2 Servings

Ingredients

1 bunch asparagus, chopped

3 cups chicken broth

Salt and pepper to taste

Pinch of cinnamon

¼ teaspoon paprika

2 eggs

¼ teaspoon salt

¼ teaspoon mustard

Salt and pepper to taste

Pinch of paprika

Instructions

Bring the chicken broth to a boil, add the asparagus, turn down heat and simmer.

Add the cinnamon and paprika and simmer for 15 minutes. Puree the soup in a food processor and add pepper and salt.

Place egg in a pan and cover with cold water then bring to a boil. Reduce the heat and simmer for 15 minutes.

Drain and cool the eggs in water then remove the shells.

Slice the eggs in half, gently remove the yolks and place in a bowl then mix with mustard and salt. Mix using a fork and fill the egg whites with the egg yolk mixture.

Tomato Feta Salad

Makes 1 Serving

1 carton heirloom tomatoes

Handful fresh basil chopped

1 cup fresh feta cheese

2 tablespoons balsamic vinegar

3 tablespoons olive oil

Salt and pepper to taste

Instructions

For the dressing, simply mix balsamic vinegar, olive oil, pepper and salt in a bowl then combine the fresh mozzarella, tomatoes and basil. Drizzle the dressing over the salad and serve.

Chicken Crockpot

Makes 3 Servings

Ingredients

3 boneless, skinless chicken breasts

3 shitake mushrooms, stems removed and sliced

1 onion, chopped

2 tablespoons ghee

¼ cup chopped fresh tarragon

5 cups chicken broth

¼ cup chopped cashews

2 bunches spinach, washed

1 tablespoon fresh thyme, chopped

Instructions

In a large pan, sauté the onion in ghee for five minutes then add the mushrooms and sauté for another three minutes. Add the chicken breasts and brown each side.

Add the herbs and broth and simmer for about two hours ensuring that the chicken is covered with liquid, adding broth when necessary.

Steam the spinach and divide between three plates. Top with chicken breasts, broth and cashews.

Turkey Burger, Mustard Greens And Feta Cheese

Makes 2 Servings

Ingredients

½ lb ground turkey

2 tablespoons crumbled feta cheese

1 bunch mustard greens, washed and chopped

3 tablespoons ground almonds

1 egg white

Pinch of cayenne

Salt and pepper to taste

Instructions

Preheat the grill. Mix the egg white, turkey, salt, almonds, pepper and cayenne and form patties.

Fill a large saucepan with water and bring to boil, add the mustard greens, reduce heat and simmer for ten minutes.

Grill the burgers for ten to fifteen minutes on each side until done. In the last few minutes of grilling, top each patty with cheese.

Drain the mustard greens, divide between the plates, top with the burgers and serve.

Tofu Wrap

Makes 2 Servings

Ingredients

½ lb tofu

1 tablespoon tamari

2 tablespoons extra virgin olive oil

1 ripe avocado

1 teaspoon lemon juice

1 garlic clove

Dash of cayenne

¼ cup chopped fresh cilantro

1 cup sunflower sprouts

1 cup grated carrots

2 low-carb tortillas

Instructions

Preheat oven to 400°F. Cut the tofu into cubes, toss in tamari and olive oil and bake for 20 minutes.

Blend the avocado, garlic, lemon juice, fresh cilantro and cayenne pepper. Spread each tortilla with the avocado mixture. Place the tofu horizontally about 2/3 towards the bottom of each tortilla. Place a line of sprouts and carrots above the tofu and role the tortillas then serve.

Grilled Salmon And Steamed Chard

Makes 2 Servings

Ingredients

2 (3- ounce) salmon fillets

2 garlic cloves, chopped

2 tablespoons extra virgin olive oil

2 tablespoons chopped fresh parsley

¼ cup lemon juice

1 bunch chard, washed, chopped and steamed

Instructions

Preheat the grill.

Rinse the fillets and pat dry then rub with garlic and olive oil. Grill the salmon for five minutes each side. Put the chard on a plate, place the salmon, pour the lemon juice, and sprinkle with parsley.

Chicken Wrap

Makes 2 Servings

Ingredients

1 boneless, skinless chicken breasts

2 low carb tortillas

1 tablespoon extra virgin olive oil

Salt and pepper

3 tablespoons chevre

¼ cup sundried tomatoes, chopped

Instructions

Preheat the grill. Rub chicken with salt, pepper and olive oil then grill the chicken for ten minutes each side or until done.

Slice the chicken, arrange on 2/3 lower part of tortilla, add tomatoes above the chicken, crumble the chevre on top and roll.

Greek Salad

Makes 2 Servings

Ingredients

Salad

2 cups washed romaine lettuce leaves, torn

½ diced tomato

½ cucumber, sliced

5 black kalamata olives

½ cup crumbled feta cheese

Red onion slices

Dressing

¼ teaspoon celery seeds

1 tablespoon balsamic vinegar

2 tablespoons olive oil

1 clove garlic pressed and minced

Instructions

Mix the salad ingredients in a bowl. Combine all the dressing ingredients in another container, cover and shake well. Pour the salad dressing over the salad and serve.

Black Bean Wrap

Makes 2 Servings

Ingredients

2 cups canned black soybeans, rinsed

2 tablespoons of olive oil

2 tablespoons of tahini

¼ teaspoon ground coriander

2 teaspoons ground cumin

2 low-carb tortillas

1 cup shredded lettuce

½ cup broccoli sprouts

1 carrot grated

1 sliced avocado

Pinch of cayenne

Salt to taste

Instructions

Mix the tahini, black beans, cumin, olive oil, coriander, cayenne and salt. Spread this mixture on the tortillas. Lay the avocado, lettuce, sprouts and carrots on the tortillas then roll and serve.

Salmon and Black bean salad

Makes 4 servings

Ingredients

3 cans salmon, drained

2 cans black beans, rinsed and drained

3 shallots, finely minced

5 stalks of celery, thinly sliced

2 bell peppers, thinly sliced

2 cloves of garlic, finely minced

1 pint tomatoes, halved

1 cucumber, halved and sliced

Zest and juice from 1 lemon

½ cup olive oil

1 teaspoon salt

1 tablespoon red wine vinegar

½ teaspoon black pepper

½ teaspoon crushed red pepper flakes

1 teaspoon dried dill

½ teaspoon ground cumin

½ teaspoon smoked paprika

Instructions

Mix the celery, garlic, shallots, tomatoes, bell peppers and cucumber and add them to a bowl with the black beans. Toss with the lemon juice, olive oil, red wine vinegar, zest, salt, black pepper, dill, cumin, paprika and red pepper flakes. Test and adjust the seasonings as needed.

Drain the cans of salmon and add the salmon to the bowl then toss to combine. Let the salad sit for an hour in the refrigerator, taste while adjusting seasonings as required then serve.

Tip: You can store this salad in the refrigerator in an airtight container for even up to four days.

Stuffed Peppers

Makes 2 Servings

Ingredients

2 large red bell peppers

8 ounces ground turkey

½ cup grated parmesan cheese

2 tablespoons olive oil

½ cup quinoa

1 medium onion, chopped

4 garlic cloves, minced

¼ cup chopped fresh basil

1 tablespoon dried thyme

6 ounces crushed tomatoes

Pinch of cayenne

Salt and pepper to taste

Instructions

Preheat the oven to 350°F. Fill a large pan ¾ full with water and bring to boil. Cut the tops of the bell pepper, remove the seeds and once the water boils, put each pepper in and cook for five minutes. After the five minutes, cool with cold water and set aside.

Sauté the onions in olive oil in a large pan. Once translucent, add the turkey and stir frequently until browned. This should take five minutes.

Add the tomatoes and other herbs and cook for around ten to fifteen minutes. Cook the quinoa according to the directions on the box.

Add the salt and pepper, cayenne, parmesan and the cooked quinoa.

Stuff each pepper with the turkey stuffing and top with more grated cheese. Bake for fifteen minutes.

Green Beans

Makes 1 Serving

Ingredients

1 cup fresh green beans, washed and snapped

1/3 cup water

¼ onion cut in half twice, lengthwise

1 tablespoon sesame seeds

2 tablespoons slivered almonds

Salt and pepper to taste

1 teaspoon sesame oil

Instructions

Place the green beans and onions in a heated pan with 1 cup of boiling water then cover and cook until crisp. This should take you around 15 minutes.

Drain and drizzle with sesame oil, sesame seeds and almonds.

Quinoa And Lentil Salad

Makes 2 Servings

Ingredients

1 cup quinoa, rinsed

1 cup lentils, rinsed

1 plum tomato, diced

3 tablespoons balsamic vinegar

1 avocado, pitted, peeled and diced

2 teaspoons salt, divided

3 tablespoons extra virgin olive oil

1 teaspoon minced cilantro

2 tablespoons lemon zest

2 teaspoons sea salt, divided

Instructions

Place lentils in a saucepan, add water to cover the lentils then stir in 1 teaspoon salt and bring to boil. Reduce to simmer and cook for around ten minutes or until tender.

As the lentils cook, cook the quinoa with the remaining salt depending on the package directions.

Once the lentils are tender, drain them and transfer to a bowl, add the quinoa and stir to mix. Let this cool. Whisk together olive oil and vinegar in a separate bowl. Add avocado and tomato to the lentil mixture then drizzle with the vinaigrette. Sprinkle with lemon zest and cilantro to serve.

Veggie Burgers

Makes 16 Mini-Patties

Ingredients

1 clove garlic, chopped

2 tablespoons canola oil

½ red bell pepper, diced

1 onion, chopped

½ cup whole raw cashews

½ yellow pepper, diced

1 teaspoon oregano

1 teaspoon paprika

1 teaspoon ground cumin

1 teaspoon salt

2 (14-ounce) black beans, drained and rinsed

2 cups breadcrumbs

Juice and zest of one lemon

1/3 cup chopped cilantro

2 eggs

Small buns

1 thinly sliced onion

2 thinly sliced Roma tomatoes

Tapenade

Instructions

Heat one tablespoon of canola oil in a large pan over medium heat. Add garlic, peppers and onions and cook while stirring frequently until the peppers and onions are soft. Stir in oregano, ground pepper, paprika, cumin and salt and cook for around one minute.

Place the sautéed onion and pepper in a food processor with beans, eggs, cashews, lemon zest, cilantro and lemon juice and pulse then add the breadcrumbs and pulse until well incorporated. Chill the mixture for 15 minutes or until firm.

Heat the remaining canola oil in a pan over medium heat then spoon mixture into the pan to form patties about ½-inch thick. Make around four to six patties ensuring not to overcrowd the pan. Cook for around 4 minutes each side.

Remove from pan and serve on the rolls topped with tapenade, red onions and tomatoes.

Dinner Recipes

Mashed Cauliflower

Makes 4 Servings

Ingredients

1 head cauliflower, leaves and stems removed and cut into quarters

½ cup green onions, thinly sliced

4 tablespoons butter

2 tablespoons sour cream

½ cup almonds, finely ground

Salt and pepper to taste

Instructions

Preheat the oven to 400°F. Boil water in a large saucepan and add the cauliflower then cook until soft. Once soft, remove the cauliflower from the water and place in a bowl. Add the sour cream, butter, salt and pepper to the cauliflower and mix using a hand mixer until smooth.

Drain the cauliflower mixture using a finely meshed strainer to get rid of any excess water. You can then mix in the green onions and nuts using your hands.

Grease a pan with butter and put the cauliflower mixture then bake for six minutes or until the cauliflower is golden on top.

Baked Halibut With Green Beans

Makes 4 Servings

Ingredients

4 (3-ounce) halibut fillets

2 garlic cloves chopped

1 lb green beans, ends snipped

5 tablespoons almonds

2 tablespoons avocado oil

2 tablespoons lemon juice

4 tablespoons chopped parsley

For the Sauce

1 cup extra virgin olive oil

2 tablespoons olive oil mayonnaise

4 tablespoons capers

5 tablespoons chopped basil

4 tablespoons chopped parsley

½ cup lemon juice

Instructions

Mix the sauce ingredients in a blender and process. Preheat the oven to 400°F. Place the fish in a shallow glass bowl, pour the sauce over the fish and cover with aluminum foil. You can then bake for ten minutes or until the fish is opaque.

Fill a pan ½ full with water and boil. Reduce the heat and add the green beans then simmer for five minutes. Drain the beans well and toss in parsley, garlic, lemon juice almonds and avocado oil. Serve with the halibut.

Grilled Tuna

Makes 3 Servings

Ingredients

3 (6-ounce) tuna steaks

1 cucumber

1 head Bibb lettuce

½ chopped walnuts

5 tablespoons dulse seaweed

Marinade

1 ½ cup orange juice

4 tablespoons lime juice

3 tablespoons tamari

1 teaspoon lemon zest

Vinaigrette

3 tablespoons fresh lemon juice

¾ cup extra virgin olive oil

3 tablespoons plum vinegar

Dash of tamari

1 tablespoon chopped rosemary

Instructions

Mix the ingredients for the marinade.

Rinse the tuna steaks, dry them and place in a baking dish with the skin side up. Pour the marinade over the tuna and refrigerate for one hour.

Preheat your grill. Meanwhile, roast the walnuts in a skillet until they sizzle then allow them to cool on a plate.

Chop the cucumber into thin round slices. Place the lettuce in a bowl with the walnuts cucumber and dulse.

Mix the vinaigrette ingredients and toss with the salad before serving.

You can now grill your tuna on each side until done. This is likely to take around five minutes for each side to be done.

Baked Salmon With Asparagus

Makes 2 Servings

Ingredients

5 ounces raw salmon, cubed

½ cup chopped fresh parsley

½ cup ground walnuts

1 egg

¼ teaspoon salt

1 lb asparagus

1 teaspoon olive oil

1 tablespoon lemon juice

Sauce

1 tablespoon lemon juice

1 teaspoon capers

2 tablespoons chopped fresh dill

2 tablespoons chopped parsley

2 tablespoons mayonnaise

Instructions

Mix the salmon, parsley, walnuts, egg and salt and refrigerate for one hour.

Mix the ingredients for the sauce in a small bowl.

Chop off the ends of the asparagus. Boil water and reduce to a simmer then put the asparagus and cook for five minutes.

Form two pieces from the salmon mixture and broil the salmon mixture for five minutes each side in a greased baking dish.

Drain the asparagus and drizzle with olive oil and lemon juice and salt to taste.

Serve the baked salmon with the sauce.

Spicy Steak With Peppers

Makes 4 Servings

Ingredients

1lb. lean steak

2 tablespoons chili sauce

1 tablespoon lime juice

½ teaspoon salt, divided

½ teaspoon crushed red pepper flakes

1 green pepper, cut into strips

1 medium onion, sliced

2 teaspoons olive oil

1 medium sweet yellow pepper, sliced

1/8 teaspoon pepper

1 garlic clove, minced

1 teaspoon horseradish

¼ cup reduced fat sour cream

Instructions

Mix the limejuice, chili sauce, ¼-teaspoon salt and pepper flakes. Brush this mixture over the steak and broil for five minutes each side or until done.

Sauté the onion, yellow and green peppers in a large pan in oil until tender then add the pepper, garlic and the remaining salt then cook for another minute.

Combine the horseradish and sour cream and serve steaks with the pepper mixture and the sauce.

Grilled Lime Shrimp

Makes 2 Servings

Ingredients

6 uncooked large shrimp, peeled and deveined

3 tablespoons lime juice

1 tablespoon balsamic vinegar

2 tablespoons olive oil

1 teaspoon garlic powder

1 tablespoon Dijon mustard

Instructions

Combine the lime juice, olive oil, vinegar, mustard and garlic powder in a resealable plastic bag and add the shrimp. Seal the bag and turn to coat. Refrigerate for 1 hour while turning occasionally.

Discard the marinade and thread the shrimp onto wooden skewers. Lightly coat the grill rack with cooking oil and grill covered over medium heat for four minutes each side or until the shrimp turns pink.

Baked Tilapia With Spicy Pineapple

Makes 4 Servings

Ingredients

4 (6-ounce) fillets

¼ cup pineapple

¼ teaspoon salt

1 teaspoon chili

1 plum tomato diced

Instructions

Preheat the oven to 375°F. Line a baking sheet with aluminum foil and coat the foil with cooking spray.

Place the tilapia on the baking sheet and sprinkle some salt.

Combine the pineapple, chili and tomato in a bowl and divide the topping among the fillets.

Bake for 15 minutes or until the tilapia flakes easily when using a fork.

Broiled Scallops

Makes 2 Servings

Ingredients

1 lb scallops

6 thinly sliced bok choy

2 lime wedges

¼ cup chopped parsley

2 tablespoons chopped hazel nuts

3 tablespoons ghee

¼ teaspoon salt

Instructions

Rinse the scallops and dry. Steam the bok choy for 7 minutes.

Preheat the oven to broil. Toss the ghee, scallops and parsley in a baking dish. Broil for five minutes and serve.

Coconut Curry Chicken

Makes 2 Servings

Ingredients

2 boneless, skinless chicken breasts

1 can low-fat coconut milk

1 onion, chopped

3 garlic cloves, minced

1 tablespoon curry powder

1 bunch spinach

3 tablespoons ghee

Instructions

Sauté onion in ghee in a large pan and slice the chicken breasts diagonally. Add garlic, curry powder and 3 tablespoons of water to the pan and simmer for three minutes.

Add the chicken breasts, stir and cover and simmer for five minutes. Add the coconut milk and simmer for 20 minutes. Always ensure that the chicken is covered with the liquid.

Steam the spinach.

Serve the coconut curry chicken with the spinach.

Peppers And Turnips

Makes 2 Servings

Ingredients

2 (4-ounce) tenderloin fillets

1 red bell pepper, quartered

1 green bell pepper, quartered

3 turnips, peeled and cut into chunks

1 tablespoon butter

1 fennel root cut into half

1 tablespoon cream

Salt to taste

Dash of cinnamon

Instructions

Rub the fillets with olive oil and sprinkle with pepper and salt.

Fill a pan halfway with water, bring to boil and put the turnips and fennel. Reduce heat and simmer for 15 minutes.

Preheat the grill and fill a pan ½ full with water then bring to boil, add pepper and simmer for five minutes then remove the peppers.

Drain the fennel and turnips, put in a food processor and blend with salt, cream, cinnamon and butter.

Grill the green pepper for five minutes each side and set aside.

Grill the fillets for eight minutes on every side.

Serve the fillets with the vegetables.

Mediterranean Seafood Soup

Makes 6 Servings

Ingredients

1 lb uncooked shrimp, peeled and deveined

1 lb red snapper fillets, cut into 1-inch cubes

½ lb sea scallops

1 medium onion, chopped

1 teaspoon minced garlic, divided

1 tablespoon olive oil

¼ teaspoon crushed red pepper flakes

1 teaspoon grated lemon peel

½ lb plum tomatoes, seeded and diced

1/3 cup reduced-fat mayonnaise

½ teaspoon salt

1/3 cup minced fresh parsley

Instructions

Sauté the onion in oil in a Dutch oven until tender then add ½ teaspoon of garlic and cook for another minute. Add the lemon peel, tomatoes, pepper and stir then cook for two minutes and add the salt and bring to a boil. Reduce the heat and simmer for around ten minutes.

Add the shrimp, fish, scallops and parsley. Cover and cook for around 8 to 10 minutes. Mix the mayonnaise and remaining garlic and dollop on every serving.

Mango Barbecued Chicken

Makes 4 Servings

Ingredients

4 boneless, skinless chicken thighs

Marinade

2 tablespoons orange juice

1 ½ teaspoons olive oil

1 ½ teaspoons lime juice

1 garlic clove minced

Barbecue sauce

1 ½ teaspoons lime juice

2 tablespoons mango chutney

1 teaspoon grated orange peel

1 tablespoon minced fresh cilantro

¼ teaspoon minced ginger

1 teaspoon Dijon mustard

1 ½ teaspoons sesame seeds, toasted

Instructions

Combine the marinade ingredients in a resealable plastic bag and add the chicken. Seal the bag and turn to coat. Refrigerate for 8 hours or overnight.

For the barbecue sauce, combine the lime juice, chutney, ginger and mustard in a bowl and set aside. In another bowl, mix the sesame seeds, cilantro and orange peel and put aside.

Drain and discard the marinade. Broil chicken for 7 minutes, turn and broil the other side for six minutes. Baste chicken with half the barbecue sauce and broil for three minutes longer.

Place on a serving dish and sprinkle with the cilantro mixture. Serve with remaining sauce.

Shrimp With Garlic Sauce

Makes 4 Servings

Ingredients

1 ½ lbs. uncooked wild shrimp, peeled and deveined

2 tablespoons chili sauce

2 tablespoons tamari sauce

2 teaspoons rice wine

2 teaspoons sesame oil

3 cloves of garlic minced

1 scallion thinly sliced

Freshly cracked black pepper to taste

2 tablespoons olive oil

Instructions

Mix the tamari sauce, rice wine, chili sauce and sesame oil and put aside.

Heat olive oil in a large pan over medium heat and fry the garlic for about thirty seconds. Add the shrimp and cook both sides for about two minutes each. Add the sauce mixture and stir until the shrimp is fully coated then season with black pepper.

Remove from heat and serve with vegetables or brown rice.

Cranberry Chicken Salad

Makes 2 Servings

Ingredients

2 lbs. cooked chicken, cubed

1 cup dried cranberries

1 cup celery, diced

2/3 cup olive oil mayonnaise

2 tablespoons chopped shallot

2 tablespoons chopped tarragon

½ teaspoon black pepper

½ teaspoon salt

2 cups chopped romaine lettuce leaves

3 tablespoons white wine vinegar

Instructions

Mix all the ingredients in a bowl.

You can then serve with toasted pocket less pita wedges.

Crab Salad With Avocado And Green Beans

Makes 4 Servings

Ingredients

8 ounce cooked crabmeat

1 ½ cups green beans, end trimmed and cut into ½ inch pieces

1 avocado, peeled and cubed

½ cup Greek yogurt

2 tablespoons coarse sea salt

1 tablespoon Dijon mustard

4 tablespoons minced fresh chives

¼ teaspoon fine sea salt

1 Granny Smith Apple, peeled and cubed

Instructions

Fill a large saucepan fitted with a colander with water. Bring to a boil over high heat, add the green beans and coarse salt, and cook for three minutes or until tender.

Remove the colander from the pot, rinse beans with cold water, drain and pat dry.

Whisk mustard, fine sea salt and yogurt in a bowl. Add the green beans, avocado, chives, crabmeat and apple then toss and serve.

Rice With Grilled Shrimp

Makes 6 Servings

Ingredients

1 ¾ cups basmati rice

1 lb. shrimp, peeled and deveined

1 white onion, diced

2 tablespoons olive oil

6 cloves of garlic

2 yellow peppers, diced

2 Roma tomatoes, peeled and diced

1 teaspoon fresh ginger, minced

½ chopped parsley

3 cups water

1 cup low fat yogurt

Salt and pepper to taste

Instructions

Soak 6 wooden skewers in water for twenty minutes.

Heat olive oil in a large pan over medium heat. Add peppers and onions and cook for five minutes or until the onion is translucent.

Stir in ginger and garlic until fragrant, add the tomatoes, and mix well. Cook for around five minutes, add the rice and stir frequently until browned. Add the water and stir well to combine. Bring to a boil and reduce heat to low then cover and simmer for 15-20 minutes then remove from heat.

In a bowl, add some rice mixture to the yogurt and stir. Continue adding rice until the yogurt is warmed through then mix the entire bowl of yogurt into the rice mixture, add salt, pepper and parsley and fold to combine.

Thread 4 shrimp per skewers and then grill over medium heat for one minute each side until the shrimp is white at the center.

Juicy Turkey Burger

Makes 1 Serving

Ingredients

1 lb. ground turkey

¼ cup gouda cheese, shredded

1 cup marinara sauce

¼ cup mozzarella cheese, shredded

Salt and pepper to taste

½ cup chopped red onion

Salad greens to top burger

Whole grain burger bun

Instructions

Mix all the ingredients with the ground turkey except the greens and onion. Make 4 individual patties and grill until cooked through.

Top with salad greens and onions and serve in a bun.

Chicken With Cherry Salsa

Makes 4 Servings

Ingredients

4 boneless, skinless chicken cutlets

½ lb. cherries, pitted

1 tomato, cored and chopped

½ cup chopped white onion

½ teaspoon black pepper, divided

¾ teaspoon salt, divided

2 tablespoons chopped cilantro

2 tablespoons extra virgin olive oil

¾ cup whole wheat breadcrumbs

Instructions

Put onion, cherries, tomato, ¼ teaspoon pepper and ¼ teaspoon salt in a food processor and pulse until you have a chunky salsa.

Put breadcrumbs in a shallow dish, season the chicken with ¼ teaspoon pepper and ½ teaspoon salt then dredge in breadcrumbs to coat. Shake off the excess and discard any excess breadcrumbs.

Heat oil in a large pan over medium high heat then arrange the chicken in a single layer in a pan and cook, flipping only once until cooked and golden brown. This should take like 6-8 minutes. Transfer to plates and spoon the salsa over the top.

Desserts And Smoothies

Berries And Cream

Makes 2 Servings

Ingredients

1/3 cup blueberries

1/3 cup blackberries

1/3 cup strawberries

1/3 cup cream

Instructions

Mix berries and top with cream then serve.

Lemony Blueberry Crumble

Makes 8 Servings

Ingredients

Filling

1 teaspoon stevia

1 tablespoon lemon juice

2 packages frozen blueberries

Topping

1 cup spelt flour

Pinch of cinnamon

1 cup walnuts

3 tablespoons butter

¼ teaspoon nutmeg

Instructions

Grease a pie plate with butter.

Mix the filling ingredients and put them at the bottom of the pie plate.

Process the topping ingredients in a food processor and sprinkle topping over the blueberry filling. Bake at 350°F for 40 minutes.

Yogurt And Berries

Makes 2 Servings

Ingredients

1/3 cup blueberries

2 cups yogurt

¼ cup chopped macadamia nuts

1 teaspoon lemon juice

¼ teaspoon ground cinnamon

Instructions

Mix the blueberries, yogurt, cinnamon and lemon juice.

Sprinkle the macadamia nuts and serve.

Yogurt Parfait

Makes 2 Servings

1 cup plain yogurt

¼ cup goji berries

¼ cup raw granola (no sweetener)

Instructions

Add in the goji berries and granola to your yogurt and mix well. Put in a serving dish and top with more goji berries and granola.

Raspberry Cake

Makes 8 Servings

Ingredients

Filling

1 package silken tofu

2 tablespoons stevia

2 tablespoons lemon juice

2 small package of raspberries

Crust

½ cup almonds

½ cup cashews

Pinch of cinnamon

4 tablespoons butter

Instructions

Blend the ingredients for the filling in a blender. Blend the crust ingredients in a food processor and press on a pie plate. Pour the filling into the crust and chill for three hours then serve.

Kiwi Smoothie

Makes 1 Serving

Ingredients

2 kiwis, peeled

2 cups fresh baby spinach

½ cup water

1 carrot, peeled

1 apple, peeled and cored

1 scoop of whey protein powder

Instructions

Combine all ingredients in a blender and blend until smooth.

Pear Cantaloupe Smoothie

Makes 1 Serving

Ingredients

1 pear with skin, cored

½ medium cantaloupe, rind and seeds removed

1 cup fresh baby spinach

1 scoop whey protein powder

Ice cubes

Instructions

Mix all the ingredients in blender and blend until a smooth consistency is achieved.

Mango Delight

Makes 2 Servings

Ingredients

1 mango, peeled and chopped

1 scoop whey protein powder

1 nectarine, chopped and peeled

1 teaspoon grated lemon rind

½ cup low-fat yogurt

½ cup water

Instructions

Combine all ingredients in a blender and blend until smooth.

Tropical Delight

Makes 1 Serving

Ingredients

½ cup pineapple

½ cup coconut milk

Juice from ¼ lime

½ banana

Instructions

Combine all the ingredients in a blender and blend until smooth.

Acai Berry Banana Smoothie

Makes 1 Serving

Ingredients

3 tablespoons dried acai berries

½ banana

½ cup strawberries

½ cup almond milk

1 scoop whey protein powder

1 cup of ice

Instructions

Combine all ingredients in your blender and process until smooth.

Pear Kale Smoothie

Makes 2 Servings

Ingredients

½ pear

1 cup kale

¼ avocado

1 scoop whey protein powder

Handful of cilantro

½ lemon

½ cup coconut water

½ inch ginger

Instructions

Combine all the ingredients in a blender and blend until smooth.

Breakfast Smoothie

Makes 2 Servings

Ingredients

1/3 cup fresh berries

20 almonds

10 oz water

1 tablespoon flaxseed oil

1 scoop whey protein powder

Instructions

Combine all ingredients in a blender and blend.

Blueberry Smoothie With Almonds

Makes 2 Servings

Ingredients

½ cup frozen blueberries

2 scoops whey protein powder

¼ cup raw almonds

1 teaspoon flax oil

¼ teaspoon cinnamon

16 ounces pure water

Instructions

Combine all the ingredients in a blender and blend until smooth.

Blueberry Smoothie With Cashew Nuts

Makes 2 Servings

Ingredients

½ cup blueberries

¼ cup raw cashew nuts

2 scoops whey protein powder

Pinch of cinnamon

16 ounces of water

Instructions

Combine all ingredients in a blender and blend.

Orange Raspberry Smoothie

Makes 2 Servings

Ingredients

½ cup orange juice

1 cup raspberries

½ cup low-fat plain yogurt

½ cup water

4 ice cubes

Instructions

Add all the ingredients in a blender and blend until smooth.

Banana Mango Peach Smoothie

Makes 2 Servings

Ingredients

½ banana

½ cup fresh mango

½ cup fresh peaches

1 ½ scoops protein powder

1 cup almond milk

5 ice cubes

Instructions

Combine all ingredients in a blender and process until smooth.

Delicious Purple Smoothie

Makes 2 Servings

Ingredients

2 cups frozen blueberries

3 dates

1 scoop of whey protein powder

2 ½ cups almond milk

1 fresh purple fig

Instructions

Blend all the ingredients until smooth.

Papaya Smoothie

Makes 1 Serving

Ingredients

½ ripe papaya

1 whole lime

Vanilla extract to taste

1 cup purified water

Instructions

Combine all the ingredients in a blender and process until smooth.

Mango Ginger Smoothie

Makes 2 Servings

Ingredients

1 ripe mango

½ cup fresh orange juice

1 tablespoon fresh lime juice

1 teaspoon grated ginger

½ cup low-fat yogurt

½ cup water

Instructions

Combine all the ingredients in a blender and process until smooth.

Watermelon Ginger

Makes 1 Serving

Ingredients

1 cup watermelon, seeded and cubed

1 teaspoon lime juice

1 teaspoon grated ginger

Instructions

Blend all the ingredients until smooth.

Lemon Blueberry smoothie

Makes 2 servings

Ingredients

Juice from ½ lemon

1 cup fresh blueberries

1 cup low-fat milk

1 scoop whey protein powder

Ice cubes

Instructions

Blend all ingredients until smooth.

5 Day Meal Plan

Day 1

Breakfast

Hard boiled Eggs with Spinach

Cup of coffee or tea with a dash of stevia

Lunch

Citrus chicken Salad

Dinner

Baked Halibut with Green Beans

Dessert

Berries with yogurt

Day 2

Breakfast

Breakfast Smoothie

Lunch

Turkey Burger, Mustard Greens And Feta Cheese

Dinner

Spicy Steak with Peppers

Day 3

Breakfast

Rosemary eggs

Cup of coffee or tea with dash of stevia

Lunch

Grilled Salmon and Steamed chard

Dinner

Coconut curry chicken

Day 4

Breakfast

Avocado and Ham Scramble

Cup of green tea with dash of stevia

Lunch

Tofu Wrap

Dinner

Grilled Lime Shrimp

Dessert

A slice of Raspberry cake

Day 5

Breakfast

Mango Delight

Lunch

Baked Salmon and Asparagus

Dinner

Chicken with cherry salsa

Snacks

If you really need to eat something in between meals you can grab a handful of cashews, pecans, cashews or almonds. You can toast these nuts and mix them with some spices to make them sweeter.

You can also grab a smoothie but be careful with your fructose intake, as we do not want to overdo it.

Conclusion

When you have leptin resistance, it can be quite hard to lose weight and even if you do, you may end up adding back all the weight you may have lost thus making useless all the hard work you had put in. This leads to a cycle of losing and gaining weight. If you want to lose weight and keep off the excess weight, then you need to handle your leptin problem. You will be amazed at how losing weight will be much easier.

If you haven't already then your next step is to check out a free preview of "Leptin Resistance Revealed - The Truth About The Leptin Hormone and Obesity and How To Overcome For Permanent Weight Loss." This is the first book in Weight Loss Solution Series and is a must read if you are going on the leptin diet.

Thank you!

Sara Banks

Preview of 'Leptin Resistance Revealed'

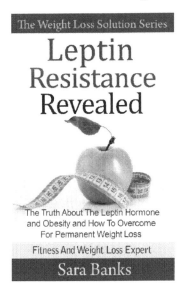

The Weight Loss Solution Series

Leptin Resistance Revealed

The Truth About The Leptin Hormone and Obesity and How To Overcome For Permanent Weight Loss

Fitness And Weight Loss Expert

Sara Banks

Leptin Resistance

As we have learned, leptin controls the amount of fat stored by signaling to the brain when you are full and do not need more food. You may then think that high leptin levels are good enough for people with obesity especially since it can control their appetite. The interesting thing is that most obese people have high levels of leptin; however, the body does not register this. This simply means that leptin has lost its ability to tell the brain that you are satisfied and that you do not need more food. Since leptin has lost its sensitivity, you will need to take more food in order to feel satisfied. Considering that leptin is usually produced by fat, you will need to eat more to have more fat stored in order for enough leptin to be produced to inform the brain that you are full and satisfied and do not need more food. This leads to a vicious cycle, which if not dealt with leads to obesity.

In order to know how to address leptin resistance, it is important that you know how it comes about. When you consume food, the body converts the food to glucose for use in body activities. Since the body can only have so much glucose, it needs to find a way of getting rid of the excess as it can easily cause hyperglycemic symptoms or vascular damage. The body stores the excess in form of fat. As I mentioned earlier, the more fat cells you have, the more leptin is produced. When you produce more leptin, the more resistance your cells become to its signal.

Causes Of Leptin Resistance

There are quite a number of things that contribute to leptin resistance. We will have a look at various things that may easily cause this resistance:

High Fructose Consumption

Fructose is sugar found mainly in fruit, table sugar and corn syrup. However, fructose in fruits is not bad as that in corn syrup and table sugar. Researchers at the University of Florida published a new journal that indicated high-fructose diets led to leptin resistance in rats and eventually triggered weight gain. During the study, rats were fed on either 60% fructose diet or fructose-free diet for a period of six months. After this period, they were then tested for leptin resistance and it was interesting to note that the rats that were on a fructose diet had leptin resistance after the six months while those who fed on a fructose-free diet had no leptin resistance. The rats on the high-fructose diets also had higher levels of triglycerides in their blood. Several studies have actually shown that higher levels of triglycerides impair the transportation of leptin to the brain thereby preventing the brain to respond to leptin adequately.

High Stress Levels

Did you know that the stress hormone cortisol causes the body to store more fat, especially in your abdominal area. Since fat cells produce leptin, the more fat you have, the more leptin you will produce making your cells resistant to leptin, which can then lead to leptin resistance. This simply means that chronic stress can easily set up a vicious cycle between cortisol production, leptin resistance and insulin resistance all, which lead to weight gain and other health problems.

Increased stress is also likely to lead to insomnia and sleep deprivation. The less sleep you get, the more leptin resistant you will be. Did you know that sleep also increases the release of a hormone called ghrelin "the hunger hormone", which then triggers hunger and increased appetite? You will then end up eating more, leading to more fat storage and hence more leptin being produced with a higher likelihood of becoming leptin resistant.

A Diet High In Simple Carbohydrates

Simple carbohydrates are like those found in highly processed foods, candy and baked foods. Simple carbohydrates are usually easily converted to glucose, which then causes a surge in the insulin levels necessitating the storage of excess sugars as fat. The more fat you have, the more leptin you will produce since leptin is produced by fat cells. Exposure to too much leptin then leads to leptin resistance where your brain can no longer hear that you are telling it to stop eating and instead burn fat. You then become hungrier leading to consumption of more simple carbohydrates and this becomes a vicious cycle.

High Insulin Levels

When you consume a meal, the pancreas releases the insulin, which is helpful in the absorption of glucose by the body cells. Without insulin, these cells cannot take up the glucose and sugar in the blood for energy. With a moderate intake in carbohydrates, the pancreas simply releases enough insulin, which then helps the muscles, liver and fat cells to take in the sugar. However, when you consume excessive amounts of carbohydrates, you end up increasing your fat since the muscle cells and liver have a limited capacity to store glucose; thus, all the excess will be sent to the fat cells for storage.

You know now what happens when you have more fat. More fat cells mean that you are likely to produce more leptin leading to high levels of leptin, which can then make the cells resistance to leptin.

Overeating

Eating more than you should even when you are supposed to stop eating can very well cause leptin resistance. When taking a meal and there is enough fat stored, leptin will be released from the adipose tissue and travel to the brain to communicate that you should stop eating. Each time you do not listen to this message, the body will have to increase leptin levels for you to hear the message. Over time, there is a lot of leptin produced to relay the message that you are satisfied. You will now actually start to eat more since it takes more leptin for you to notice that you are full. This of course leads to leptin resistance.

Too Much Exercise

Yes, too much of everything is poisonous. When on a weight loss journey, you may decide to reduce your calorie intake and increase the amount of calories you burn. You may then achieve some weight loss. However, over time, as you lose more weight and exercise, the amount of calories you burnt for instance when doing a 30-minute cardio workout will reduce since your body will adapt. It is during this time that most people experience some sort of weight plateau where they no longer lose any weight. What do many people do in such instances? The answer is simple; they turn to reducing their calorie intake further and increasing the amount of exercise. This puts unnecessary strain on the body, which in turn makes it respond by releasing the stress hormone, cortisol, because you are under pressure.

Consumption Of Lectins

You may have heard of some people not eating grains and other foods rich in lectins because of different reasons. Lectins usually bind to the intestinal lining, in particular the villi of the small intestine, where nutrients flow into before they can cross into the bloodstream. Once the lectins damage the villi, your body is unable to digest and absorb the nutrients from the small intestines. This damage may also encourage parasites and other pathogenic organisms and eventually lead to leaky gut syndrome where the intestinal lining has open gaps where the lectins and other organisms can get directly into the bloodstream. Lectins usually have a high affinity for leptin receptors and it is actually believed that they can desensitize these receptors leading to the production of more leptin in order for the brain to get the message. This eventually leads to leptin resistance.

Symptoms Of Leptin Resistance

Would you want to know if you have a leptin problem, which is making it hard for you to lose weight? We will have a look at some of the common symptoms of leptin resistance in order for you to try to find out if you have a leptin resistance so that you can take the right steps to deal with the situation at hand.

An Increased Appetite And Cravings

Leptin works to decrease appetite. When you have had enough to eat, your fat cells will release leptin, which will dull your appetite by informing the brain that it is time to stop eating since you have enough fat reserves. However......

Check Out My Other Books

Below you'll find some of my other books that are popular on Amazon and Kindle as well. You can visit my author page on Amazon to see other work done by me.

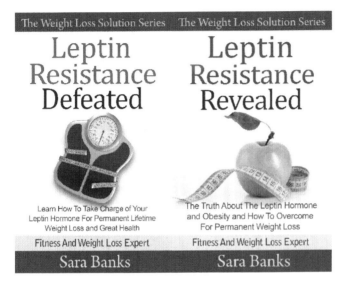

This document is geared towards providing exact and reliable information in regards to the topic and issue covered. The publication is sold with the idea that the publisher is not required to render accounting, officially permitted, or otherwise, qualified services. If advice is necessary, legal or professional, a practiced individual in the profession should be ordered.

- From a Declaration of Principles which was accepted and approved equally by a Committee of the American Bar Association and a Committee of Publishers and Associations.

In no way is it legal to reproduce, duplicate, or transmit any part of this document in either electronic means or in printed format. Recording of this publication is strictly prohibited and any storage of this document is not allowed unless with written permission from the publisher. All rights reserved.

The information provided herein is stated to be truthful and consistent, in that any liability, in terms of inattention or otherwise, by any usage or abuse of any policies, processes, or directions contained within is the solitary and utter responsibility of the recipient reader. Under no circumstances will any legal responsibility or blame be held against the publisher for any reparation, damages, or monetary loss due to the information herein, either directly or indirectly.

Respective authors own all copyrights not held by the publisher.

The information herein is offered for informational purposes solely, and is universal as so. The presentation of the information is without contract or any type of guarantee assurance.

The trademarks that are used are without any consent, and the publication of the trademark is without permission or backing by the trademark owner. All trademarks and brands within this book are for clarifying purposes only and are the owned by the owners themselves, not affiliated with this document.

42258474R00049

Made in the USA
Lexington, KY
14 June 2015